YOGA FOR MALE

An Effective Guide to Improve Performance, Increase Flexibility and Build Strength

STEPHENIE DEAN

TABLE OF CONTENT

CHAPTER 1

INTRODUCTION

Male yoga practitioner's square measure referred to as yogis and feminine yoga practitioners square measure referred to as yoginis. Each practiced and schooled yoga long before any written record of yoga came into existence.

Over future 5 millennia, yogis passed the discipline all the way down to their students, and plenty of totally different colleges of yoga developed because they apply swollen its international reach and recognition.

The "Yoga Sanskrit literature," a 2,000-year-old piece of writing on yogistic philosophy by the Indian sage Patanjali, could be a handbook on a way to master the mind, management the emotions, and grow spiritually. The Yoga Sanskrit literature is that the earliest written account of yoga and one among the oldest texts living and provides the framework for all trendy yoga.

Yoga is standard for its postures and poses, however they weren't a key a part of original yoga traditions in Asian nation. Fitness wasn't a primary goal. Practitioners and followers of yogistic tradition centered instead on different practices, like increasing non secular energy mistreatment respiration ways and mental focus.

The tradition began to achieve quality within the West at the top of the nineteenth century. Associate explosion of interest in bodily property yoga occurred within the Twenties and Thirties, initial in Asian nation and later within the West.

CHAPTER 2

WHAT IS YOGA

Yoga simply means union. Etymologically, it's connected to land word, yoke. Yoga means that union with God, or, union of the insufficient, ego-self with the divine Self, the infinite Spirit.

Most people within the West, and conjointly several in Asian nation, confuse yoga with yoga, the system of bodily postures.

However yoga is primarily a religious discipline.

Not that there's something wrong with active yoga. The body could be a part of our attribute, and should be unbroken match thus it doesn't impede our religious efforts. However, those that are centered on fulfillment don't essentially have to follow it the maximum amount or in the slightest degree.

Hatha Yoga is that the physical branch of Raja Yoga, actuality science of yoga. Raja Yoga could be a system of meditation techniques that facilitate to harmonize human consciousness with the divine consciousness.

Yoga is AN art yet as a science. It a science, as a result of it offers sensible strategies for dominant body and mind, thereby creating deep meditation attainable. And it's an art, for unless it's practiced intuitively and sensitively it'll yield solely superficial results.

Yoga isn't a system of beliefs. It takes under consideration the influence on one another of body and mind, and brings them into mutual harmony. So often, for example, the mind cannot concentrate just because of tension or ill health within the body, that forestall the energy from flowing to the brain. So often, too, the energy within the body is weakened as a result of the need is dispirited or unfit by harmful emotions.

Yoga works primarily with the energy within the body, through the science of pranayama, or energy-control. Prana means that conjointly 'breath.' Yoga teaches however, through breath-control, to still the mind and attain higher states of awareness.

The higher teachings of yoga take one on the far side techniques, and show the yogi, or yoga professional person, the way to direct his energy in such how as not solely to harmonize human with divine consciousness, however to merge his consciousness within the Infinite.

The ordinary person's energy is fast in his body. The shortage of accessibility of that energy to his can prevents him from affectionate the Lord one-pointedly with any of the 3 alternative aspects of his nature: heart, mind, or soul. Only if the energy is withdrawn from the body and directed upward in deep meditation is true inner communion attainable.

Yoga could be a terribly ancient science; it's thousands of years previous. The perceptions derived from its follow kind the backbone of the greatness of Asian nation, which for hundreds of years has been legendary. The truths espoused within the yoga teachings; however, don't seem to be restricted to Asian nation, nor to those that consciously follow yoga techniques. Several saints of alternative religions conjointly, together with several Christian saints, have discovered aspects of the religious path that are intrinsic to the teachings of yoga.

CHAPTER 3

UNDERSTANDING SOME BASIC TYPES OF YOGA

Modern yoga has evolved with attention on exercise, strength, flexibility, and respiratory. It will facilitate boost physical and mental well being.

There square measure several kinds of yoga, and no vogue is additional authentic or superior to a different. The secret's to settle on a category applicable for your fitness level.

Types and designs of yoga might include:

Bikram yoga: Additionally referred to as "hot" yoga, Bikram happens in by artificial means heated rooms at temperatures of nearly a hundred and five degrees and forty percent humidness. It consists of twenty six poses and a sequence of 2 respiratory exercises.

Ashtanga yoga: It entails or uses ancient yoga teachings. It became well-liked throughout the 70s. Ashtanga applies six established sequences of postures that chop-chop link each movement thereto breath.

Jivamukti yoga: Once you point out Jivamukti it merely suggests that "liberation whereas living." this kind emerged in 1984 and incorporates religious teachings and practices that concentrate on the fast flow between poses instead of the poses themselves.

Hatha yoga: this will be categorized as a generic term for any variety of yoga that teaches physical postures.

Iyengar yoga: It focuses on finding the right alignment in every cause employing a varying of props, like blocks, blankets, straps, chairs, and bolsters.

This is known as vinyasa. Every category contains a theme, which is explored through yoga scripture, chanting, meditation, asana, pranayama, and music. Jivamukti yoga may be physically intense.

Kripalu yoga: It merely teaches practitioners to grasp, accept, and learn from the body. A student of Kripalu learns to seek out their own level of apply by trying inward. The categories sometimes begin with respiratory exercises and mild stretches, followed by a series of individual poses and final relaxation.

Kundalini yoga: Kundalini suggests that "coiled, sort of a snake." Kundalini yoga could be a system of meditation that aims to unleash repressed energy.

A class usually begins with vocalizing and ends with singing. In between, it options posture, pranayama, and meditation tailored to form a selected outcome.

Power yoga: within the late 80s, practitioners developed this active and mesomorphy of yoga, supported the standard ashtanga system.

Sivananda: This can be a system supported a five-point philosophy. This philosophy maintains that correct respiratory, relaxation, diet, exercise, and positive thinking work along to create a healthy Hinduism life-style. Usually uses a similar twelve basic posture, bookended by sun salutations and savasana poses.

Viniyoga: once you point out Viniyoga we are saying it will adapt to a person, in spite of ability. Viniyoga lecturers need in-depth coaching and have a tendency to be specialists on anatomy and yoga medical care.

Yin: This can be a quiet, reflective yoga apply, additionally known as Taoist yoga. Rule yoga permits the discharge of tension in key joints, including:

The ankles

Knees

Hips

The whole back

Neck

Shoulders

Yin poses square measure passive, which means that gravity shoulders most of the force and energy.

Prenatal yoga: ante partum yoga uses postures that practitioners have designed for those that square measure pregnant. It will support individuals in obtaining into form once gestation similarly as supporting health throughout gestation.

Restorative yoga: this can be a calming technique of yoga. someone spends a restorative yoga category in four or 5 straightforward poses, victimization props like blankets and bolsters to sink into deep relaxation while not exerting any

effort in holding the cause.

CHAPTER 4

STEPS TO KNOW IN CARRYING OUT YOGA PRACTICE

I. **Choose a focus to practice yoga:**

Before beginning yoga, it will facilitate to work out why you would like to apply. Yoga is a way of physical exertion, the way to scale back and manage stress, a method of healing associated un-wellness or injury, or a path to non secular fulfillment and peace.

Accept that parts of wellbeing you would like to figure on, like strength, flexibility, stamina, anxiety, and depression. You may additionally need to apply for your general well-being.

Take into account writing down your focus for your apply. Update it often and revise it as you become a lot of at home with yoga and grow as a student.

For instance, you may have a goal like "I need to apply for a minimum of five minutes each day or I need to create enough strength to an arm balance posture like Lolasana.

II. **Take note that there is no such thing as right or good yoga:**

There are altogether totally different styles and ways in which during which to look at yoga and there'll endlessly be felt yoga practitioners than you. It's important to remember that yoga is neither a contest nor a customary sport, but a non-public observes of attentiveness, relaxation, and disposition that are meant to enhance your life and body. There isn't any right or wrong because of do yoga. Your observation got to be concerning your journey first and foremost.

Anyone can observe and have the advantage of yoga. Group action yoga into your routine can facilitate improve your physical and psychological state, though you merely observe for 10 minutes day by day.

It'll take some time to look out a specific vogue or school of yoga you fancy. Similarly, finding the right teacher for you and your goals can take some trial and error.

Observe keeping associate degree open mind and adopt a non-judgmental angle.

Bear in mind that there is no competition in yoga. One and everyone have altogether totally different skills and additionally the goal of yoga is to specialize in you, not what others do.

III. Bring all equipment you may want to practice with:

All you really ought to follow yoga is that the ability to

breathe. Sure items of apparatus might assist you feel more leisurely, though, particularly within the starting. Think about having props like a yoga belt, yoga block, and an outsized blanket or bolster, too. These items of apparatus will facilitate improve and deepen your yoga follow likewise as creating it more leisurely.

Search for a mat that's padded which encompasses a non-slippery end. If you're on a budget, you'll perpetually use a blanket, towel, or couch cushions to feature a touch of additional comfort rather than shopping for a replacement mat.

You'll obtain mats and props at sports equipment stores, yoga studios, or at on-line yoga retailers.

IV. Put on a comfortable cloth that will enable you move freely:

You'll want covering that's comfy and breathes simply. This may assist you higher bring home the bacon a full vary of motion and adaptability and conjointly keep you from tugging at too tight covering.

You don't essentially would like special yoga covering; however attempt carrying one thing comfy that does not prohibit your movement. Girls will wear leggings, a tank top, and a sports bandeau. Men will wear a combine of athletic shorts and a tee shirt.

As you are trying a lot of advanced poses you'll need tighter pants and shirts that will not fall or move, distracting you within the method.

If you're doing Bikram yoga, that takes place in a very heated space, or athletically intense yoga like Jivamukti, check that to wear light-weight, breathable covering that absorbs sweat.

V.   Get a comfortable spot to practice:

If you've set to relinquish yoga a attempt reception before reaching to a category, notice a cushy and quiet house during which to explore your yoga follow. Certify you've got many area to maneuver and in some manner to shut yourself off to the skin world.

You'll want a couple of inches on either side of your mat so you don't run into a wall or the rest.

 Certify the place you follow is quiet and calm so nobody will disturb your focus. You'll additionally need somewhere that's comfortable: a moist and chilly basement might not be the most effective choice

VI. Do a gradual warming up with sun salutation:

Yoga may be quite active; therefore it's vital to heat up your body properly. Doing a number of rounds of sun salutations, or Surya Namaskar, will effectively prepare your muscles and mind to observe yoga.

There are 3 totally different variations of sun salutations. Do 2-3 rounds of Surya Namaskar A,

B, and C to heat up. These totally different sun salutations will interact and condition your muscles and may facilitate guarantee a secure and a lot of pliable observe.

Flow categories can usually begin with a sun salutation preparation. Active these reception could assist you feel lighter for after you conceive to be part of a category.

VII. Take note regarding a few yoga asanas:

There square measure a large type of yoga poses, or asanas, that one will observe and those they vary from troublesome and strenuous to easy and quiet. Begin your yoga observes by learning a number of asanas that you just will relish, feel snug execution, and that additionally suit your yoga goals. Hold every attitude for 3-5 breaths.

There square measure four differing kinds of yoga pose: standing poses, inversions, backbends, and forward bends. attempt one or 2 from every sort to balance your observe.

Standing causes embrace mountain pose (Tadasana), tree cause (Vrksasana), and also the individual Series (Virabhadrasana I, II, and III).

Inversions embrace downward-facing dog (Adho Mukha

Svanasana), dolphin cause, gymnastic exercise (Mukha Vrksasana), and acrobatic feat (Salamba Sirsasana).

Backbends embrace locust cause (Salabhasana), elapid cause (Bhujangasana), and bridge cause (Setu Bandha Sarvangasana).

 You'll add a twisting attitude to neutralize and stretch your spine between backbends and forward bends if you wish. Twisting causes embrace Bharadvaja's twist (Bharadvajasana) or 0.5 lord of the fishes pose (Ardha Matsyendrasana).

Forward folds embrace seated forward bend (Paschimottanasana) and star cause (Tarasana), which may be a wide-legged forward fold.

Finish your observation by holding remains cause (Savasana) for 3-5 minutes. This could facilitate stabilize your systema nervosum and management bodily stress.

Invariably balance out asanas that favor one aspect by doing them on the alternative aspect.

VIII. Take full control of your breath:

Yogic respiration, or pranayama, is one in every of the core skills of any yoga observe. Specializing in your respiration will deepen your posture observe, tune you into your own body, and permits you to relax.

 Pranayama will facilitate your body distribute atomic number 8 to its totally different components. The goal is to breathe deeply by eupnoea and eupnoea fully and during a balanced manner through your nose. As an example, you'd inhale for four breaths, hold for two counts, and so exhale fully for four breaths. You'll be able to vary the counts consistent with your skills.

If you would like to induce the foremost out of your Hinduism respiration, therefore sit upright, together with your shoulders back to permit for the total capability of breath. Breathe slowly and equally by focusing from your abdomen, pull in your belly to expand your lungs and skeletal structure.

You'll be able to conjointly attempt Ujjayi respiration, which may assist you flow through your observe additional effectively. You are doing Ujjayi respiration by eupnoea and eupnoea equally through your nose and creating a small sound just like the ocean once you breathe.

IX. Carryout yoga practice daily:

No matter what Asanas, Pranayam, or goals you select for

your yoga observe, it helps to observe as typically as you'll be able to. Although you'll be able to solely spare 10-15 minutes, then a lot of typically you observe, the a lot of you'll be able to learn and reap the advantages of yoga.

CHAPTER 5

POSSIBLE RISK AND SIDE EFFECT

Yoga is low-impact and safe for individuals once a well-trained tutor or instructor is guiding the follow.

Injury because of yoga is occasional barrier to continuing follow, and severe injury because of yoga is rare. However, think about a number of factors before beginning.

Anyone that is pregnant or has an ongoing medical condition, like high vital sign, glaucoma, or neuralgia, ought to seek advice from their attention professional person before active yoga. They will have to be compelled to alter or avoid some yoga poses.

Beginners ought to avoid extreme poses and troublesome techniques, like acrobatic feat, position, and forceful respiratory.

When victimization yoga to manage a condition, don't replace standard medical aid with yoga or table seeing an attention supplier concerning pain or the other medical downside.

THE END